Bodyweight Training For Women:

Bodyweight Training and Exercise Handbook

By

Charles Maldonado

Table of Contents

Introduction 5

Chapter 1. What is a Bodyweight Training?.......................... 7

Chapter 2. The Benefits of Bodyweight Exercises for Women
.... 8

Chapter 3. Types of Bodyweight Exercises for Women 14

    Common Core Bodyweight Exercises 15

    Common Upper Body Bodyweight Exercises.................. 19

    Common Lower Body Bodyweight Exercises 22

Chapter 4. Bodyweight Workout Example......................... 25

Chapter 5. Bodyweight Training Is Ideal for Women of All Ages.. 29

Thank You Page 31

Bodyweight Training For Women: Bodyweight Training and Exercise Handbook

By Charles Maldonado

© Copyright 2015 Charles Maldonado

Reproduction or translation of any part of this work beyond that permitted by section 107 or 108 of the 1976 United States Copyright Act without permission of the copyright owner is unlawful. Requests for permission or further information should be addressed to the author.

This publication is designed to provide accurate and authoritative information in regard to the subject matter covered. This work is sold with the understanding that the publisher is not engaged in rendering legal, accounting, or other professional services. If legal advice or other expert assistance is required, the services of a competent professional person should be sought.

First Published, 2015

Printed in the United States of America

Introduction

For women who are looking to live a life of great health and vitality, there are unfortunately no shortcuts, magic wands or sure-fire recipes that will accomplish these goals in a realistic and effective manner. While a proper diet and nutrition is an essential building block to a women's overall good health, engaging in a regular exercise regimen or some form of physical activity is an excellent way in which women can achieve a sound body and mind. Regular exercise not only gives the potential to live longer and healthier life, but also improves mood and memory, helps manage weight and prevent weight gain and can help prevent the onset of many diseases.

While the benefits of exercise for women are numerous and essential, finding ways to get much-needed and regular physical activity can be easier said than done. The modern woman juggles many responsibilities in regards to their careers and families, and getting into the gym is sometimes that last thing on their minds. For many women who desire to adopt a regular exercise regimen that is versatile, highly adaptable and able to fit into their busy family and work lives becomes paramount. If you are a women looking for that ideal exercise program that can be done anywhere and anytime with the minimum of equipment and hassle, bodyweight training will satisfy all of those needs and provide you with a body that looks great and feels even better.

Chapter 1. What is a Bodyweight Training?

Bodyweight training is a strength-based exercise program that involves the use of your own body weight to provide resistance that helps build and tone muscle. Bodyweight training does not require the use of free weights or the use of exercise machines, you only need to start off with a few basic exercises and have ample space to perform these exercises. Since machines or weights aren't required, you can engage in bodyweight training anywhere and at any time. Whether it is in the living room, your bedroom, the office, the hotel or at a local park, bodyweight training is highly versatile and adaptable to any situation.

Chapter 2. The Benefits of Bodyweight Exercises for Women

For women who are looking to build a lean and toned physique, they may not think that it is possible to accomplish those goals without the use of free weights or special exercise machines. Far too often, women may be hesitant in adopting an exercise programs because exercise itself is made out to be a difficult, scientific endeavor that involves many hours in the gym and many complex movements. Additionally, many women may abandon their current workout regimens after a short period of time because of extreme fatigue or injury. Bodyweight exercises are a great way for women to get introduced into the world of regular physical activity because it not only helps build muscle, bodyweight exercises also improve overall cardiovascular health.

The following are a few of the benefits that women can enjoy employing a bodyweight exercise program:

Bodyweight Training is Judgment Free

Many women may shy away from the gym because of the thought that other people may judge them in how they do exercises. With bodyweight training, women can engage in exercise in the comfort of their home. Women can listen to their inner dialogue and push themselves as hard as they want to and are able to realistically challenge themselves. Women are also able to take a step back and evaluate their progress and make adjustments to their routines. Additionally, women can take part in bodyweight training with friends in a fun environment.

Bodyweight Training Shows You How Your Body Moves

Building functional strength requires the body to be able to engage in a full range of motion. Using free weights, machines and other apparatus have a limited range of motion, which can increase the risk of injury. With full of range of motion that is possible with bodyweight training, your joints can move more freely which helps improve posture, balance and overall strength. Additionally, these exercises can also be used to rehabilitate workout-related injuries.

Bodyweight Training is Efficient

Since there is no equipment that needs to be used, bodyweight exercises are extremely efficient and woman can quickly move from one exercise to another. The quick transitions and shorter rest periods, allow women to raise their heart rate and burn calories faster. An additional benefit of bodyweight training for women is the fact they can get two workouts in one. Bodyweight exercises are able to provide both strength training and cardiovascular fitness in a workout program that can benefit anybody, even if time is short. For example, women can perform a series of push-ups then in the next exercise perform a set of jumping jacks then can incorporate reverse flyes using water bottles or other household items. With the great variety of exercises, women can easily mix and match their exercises and workout to change both pace and intensity.

Bodyweight Exercises are Easy to Modify

No matter a women's age, fitness level or limitations, bodyweight exercises can be modified to fit anyone. Those who are beginning a bodyweight exercise program can start off with exercises with low repetitions and can increase those repetitions as they begin to build strength. For example, women can start off by performing kneeling push-ups and can graduate to regular push-ups once their strength increases. Additionally, women can also vary the difficulty of their workouts by performing exercises at a slower pace, and by employing perfect technique.

Bodyweight Exercises Can Be Done Anywhere and at Anytime

Many women have busy schedules in which they are juggling many responsibilities with the careers and families, so devoting the time needed to properly exercise is at a premium. Bodyweight exercises can be performed anywhere and anytime, and these exercises can be performed without machines or other equipment, and can be a great form of stress release that can be done at home, office, hotel room or anywhere else there is space.

Bodyweight Exercises Can Be Done at Little to No Cost

If women opt to use more traditional routes of exercise it can have the potential to be an expensive endeavor. Both gym memberships and personal trainers can be costly and significantly impact household and personal budgets. Bodyweight exercises have become increasingly popular among women because of their simplicity and there is no need for equipment. If equipment is needed, women can often use household items such as water bottles or milk jugs.

Bodyweight Exercises are Safe

Injury due to exercise is among the most common reasons why women abandon their regular workouts. While the common saying that *no pain no gain* may hold true in the world of fitness, the aches and pains associated with exercise can turn many people away. Bodyweight exercises are relatively safe for men and women of all fitness levels and experience. In fact, the basic movements of bodyweight exercises can not only prevent injury, but can also be used to rehabilitate any injury.

Bodyweight Exercises Provide a Great Variety of Movements

Exercises such as rows and dumbbell curls can be boring and women can quickly lose interest in their workout routines. With bodyweight exercises, there are countless variations to spice up workouts and provide new challenges that can be exciting. Basic moves such as sit-ups, push-ups and lunges can be easily modified and can provide women with a great variety of movement to incorporate into their bodyweight workouts. With the variety of exercises that are possible, bodyweight training can also help break through any plateaus and will help women continually progress in both increasing strength and stamina.

Bodyweight Exercises Provide Results

Bodyweight exercises can provide excellent and measurable results for women. These results are possible because the exercises that are found in bodyweight training are comprised of what are called *compound movements*. Compound movements involve the movement of numerous joints and muscles. Simple exercises such as push-ups and chin-ups are some of the most effective exercises people can do to increase strength. These exercises strength one's core, which are the group of muscles centered in a person's midsection and pelvic regions. Strengthening the core will lead to improvements in strength throughout the entire body.

Chapter 3. Types of Bodyweight Exercises for Women

Bodyweight exercises can be separated those exercises that target the upper body, lower body and the important core muscles of the abdominal and pelvic areas. While certain exercises target specific areas of the body, they can be easily modified and combined with other exercises in order for women to achieve for a full-body workout. These exercises can also be easily modified to be made easier for the beginner, and with subtle changes, more repetitions and slower cadences the exercises can be made more challenging for those who have advanced levels of fitness.

With the wide variety of bodyweight exercises, there are limitless combinations of workouts that women can choose from when they design their own workout routines. Additionally, these workouts can be done with a group of friends, which can add to the enjoyment of bodyweight training and can provide women with an enjoyable form of motivation. The following are some of the many examples of bodyweight exercises that women can utilize for their own bodyweight workouts.

Common Core Bodyweight Exercises

It is important for women to understand that thorough and proper exercise of their core muscles is an extremely important facet of bodyweight training. The core is a series of muscles that are an integral part in almost every body movement. When it is said that exercises are "working the core", they are working the muscle in the pelvis, abdominal and back muscles. When women have strength in their core muscles, it improves balance and coordination, improves flexibility, and will help with posture and will help women breathe much easier. Most importantly, strong core muscles help women improve their overall strength in the rest of their bodies.

1. Planks—planks are one of the most basic exercises women can utilize to help strengthen their core. To execute the plank, women will place their forearms on the ground and place their toes on the floor. It is important that the torso is straight and rigid and the body forms a straight line all the way from the head to the toes with no bending. The position is held as long as possible as the head is relaxed and looking forward. The basic plank position can be modified in a number

of ways. For example, women can lift a leg in the air, use a small bench, or use an exercise ball in order to increase intensity, difficulty and to work different muscle groups to burn more calories

2. Side Planks—when women perform a side plank, they begin with lying on their side and positioning their elbow just under the shoulder. With the elbow in place, women would then lift themselves off the floor while being sure their body remains rigid and stiff. In general, the side plank position will be hold up to a count of ten then may switch sides. As with the regular plank, the side plank can be modified for intensity by lifting the top leg as high as possible. Additionally, women can also use their hand instead of their elbow in order to prop themselves up.

3. Push-ups—push-ups are arguably the most basic exercise movement. While the push-up is basic, it provides women with an effective workout for multiple body parts, including their core muscles. When done correctly, push-ups not only effectively work the core, but also the upper body parts such as triceps, shoulders, and the chest. Additionally, properly done push-ups are excellent leg workouts. In order for push-

ups to be an effective core workout, it is very important that women use perfect form.

For the basic push-up, it starts with getting on the floor and positioning the hands slightly wider than the shoulders. Women will then raise their toes to keep balanced and must remember to keep their body in a straight line. When women lower themselves the abs and core muscles must be tightened by pulling the belly button towards the spine. It is also important for women to inhale as they lower themselves to the ground and exhale when they return to the starting position.

Additionally, the elbows must be at a 90 degree angle when people are at their lowest point in the push-up. Women can add elements to the basic push-up in order to increase strength and intensity. Women can use an exercise or medicine ball, change the width of the arms and hands, and can even incorporate a dumbbell or other weighted object.

4. Crunches—crunches start with a women lying on their back with knees bent and feet planted on the floor. Their hands are placed behind their head and they will slowly lift their head and shoulders from the

floor. Once the upper part of the back has cleared the ground, they will slowly work their way back down to the original laying position. It is important that the core muscles are engaged when performing a crunch.

5. Flutter Kicks—for this movement, women will lie on their back with their arms at their sides and their palms facing downward. As the legs are extended outward, women will then lift their heels so they are about six inches off the ground. While engaging the core muscles, women will make quick pulsating movement with their legs.

6. V-Sits--To perform this exercise, women need to start in a seated position and lift their legs to a 45 degree angle. As the legs are raised, the arms must be placed straight forward and extend towards the shins. While the position is held, good posture must be maintained for proper form. When going back to normal seated position, women need to try and hold the position just before the legs and hands make contact with the floor.

Common Upper Body Bodyweight Exercises

1. Donkey Kick—women will start in the push-up position with their legs together. As they engage their core muscles, they will kick both legs in the air with their knees bent. When performing the donkey kick, women should try to hit their glutes. It is also important that women try to land as gently as possible when returning to the push-up position.

2. Triceps Dip—women will be seating on the ground facing front with their knees slightly bent in front of a chair or small bench. They will grab the edge of the chair or bench and straighten their arms. The arms should be bent at a 90 degree angle while going upward, then straightened on the downward motion. Once strength has been built, women can increase the intensity of this exercise by reach out one arm while lifting the opposite leg.

3. Inchworm—this exercise is excellent for women to build upper body strength. Additionally, the inchworm is considered a plyometric exercise which builds explosiveness. They will need to stand as tall as possible and reach towards the floor with their

fingertips. Keeping the legs as straight as possible without locking, they can slowly lower the torso and walk their hands forward as they do so. Once people achieve a push-up like position, they can take small steps until their feet and hands meet.

4. Reverse Flys—Women can use dumbbells or household items such as bottles of water or other items that have some weight. To start this exercise, women will stand up straight and place one foot slightly in front of the other. With abdominal muscles engaged and with palms facing forward, women will bend slightly forward at the waist and extend their arms out to the side while squeezing the shoulder blades.

5. Shoulder Stabilizers—Women will start this exercise lying on their stomach. The arms will be extended upward and the palms will be facing inward. Women will move then move their arms to form the shapes of letters, such as V, I, T and O as examples. It is important to move slowly between the formations of each letter.

6. Diamond Push-ups—as stated in the core exercise section, push-ups are an excellent all-around

bodyweight exercise. An excellent push-up variation that provides an excellent workout for the triceps is the diamond push-up. With this push-up, women place their hands so that their index fingers and thumbs touch. This provides the base where women can push upward.

Common Lower Body Bodyweight Exercises

1. Lunges—lunges are a basic bodyweight exercise that women can perform that are excellent in building strength in their leg muscles. They will start with their hands placed on their hips and their feet placed shoulder-width apart. With one leg placed forward, they will slowly lower themselves until the forward knee is either close to touching the ground or placed at a 90 degree angle. People then return to the starting position, switch legs then repeat the motion.

As with the other basic movements, women can add variations to the lunge to make them more challenging. For instance, women can perform jump lunges where jump explosively in the air as they switch legs. Additionally, women can do walking lunges where they start in normal lunge position with their knees touching or almost making contact with floor. Women will then alternate legs and bring their alternate leg forward in a walking motion without pause.

2. Wall Sits—this exercise is another staple movement for women who perform bodyweight training. To effectively perform the wall sit, women starts by

leaning against a wall and slowly lower themselves until their thighs reach parallel to the ground. The knees must be directly above the ankles and the back must be kept straight. If possible, this seated position should be held for one minute, but beginners or others with limitations can perform this exercise for shorter durations.

3. Squats—another staple lower body exercise in bodyweight training, women will stand with their feet shoulder-width apart with their arms relaxed at the sides of the body. Additionally, their toes should also be pointed outward at a slight angle. Women will then pull back shoulders and bend at the knees while both the butt and hips are pushed forward. To effectively perform this exercise, it is important for women to keep the weight on the heels and try to get the thighs parallel to the ground if possible.

4. Step-Ups—by using a small step stool, bench or finding a set of stairs, women will place their right foot on the elevated surface. They will then step up until the leg is straight and then will return to resting position. For beginners, they should focus on doing 10

repetitions per side to start then increase repetitions as they gain strength.

5. Calf Raises—from the standing position, rise up to the front and balls of the toes and try to keep the knees straight and the heels off of the floor. Women want to hold that position as long as possible, then slowly return to the resting position. Women can utilize an inclined surface such as steps to increase the intensity of the movement. Additionally, the use of lighter dumbbells or other household items can help increase strength and work other muscle groups.

6. Single Leg Deadlifts—women start in a standing position with their feet placed together. The right leg starts to lift slowly and the arms and torso lower. To complete the exercise, women will slowly raise up back into standing position. This exercise can be scaled to fit beginners with assistance from a chair or bench. With increased strength, people can try to lower themselves as close to the ground as possible.

Chapter 4. Bodyweight Workout Example

With the basic exercises and movements outlined above, women can design a bodyweight workout that is unique to their needs and their schedule. For those women who claim they have no time for a workout, an effective bodyweight workout can take as little as 15-20 minutes a day. These bodyweight workouts can be done anywhere and at any time, whether it is during a lunch hour, in a local park on a sunny afternoon or in the comfort of a living room.

The Importance of the Warming Up and Cooling Down

Before you begin your workout, it is very important to thoroughly warm up your muscles. Getting the heart rate elevated and the blood and oxygen flowing through your muscles greatly reduces the chances for injury. If you happen to be running short on time, you always want to cut short the actual workout AND NOT THE WARMUP. It is equally important to slowly and carefully stretch after your workout as you cool down. Women should perform bodyweight training two to three times weekly on non-consecutive days. Rest days allow muscles to repair and rest will help build muscle.

An Example of an Easy Bodyweight Workout for Women

The following is an example of a basic bodyweight workout that women can use. With each exercise, it is important to not there is no rest periods in between each exercise.

*Jumping Jacks (30 seconds)

*Prisoner Squats (20 repetitions—this squat variation involves placing hands behind the head)

*Basic Push-ups (20 repetitions)

*Walking Lunges (12 repetitions each side)

*Mountain Climbers (10 repetitions each side—this move starts in pushup position and women alternates raising their knees to their chest)

*Inverted Hamstring (8 repetitions each side—women start in standing position and slowly raise one leg while leaning forward, ensuring they keep their back and leg in a straight line as they bend)

*T-Stabilization (8 repetitions per side—starting in push-up position, women will shift their weight to one arm while lifting the opposite arm into the air)

*Jogging in Place (30 seconds)

This circuit should be repeated up to five times if at all possible. Beginners may have to limit the number of circuits until their strength and stamina improve. Many of these exercises can be interchangeable or replaced with other exercises to increase intensity and to burn more calories.

Don't Forget Proper Diet and Nutrition

In order for an exercise program to be truly effective, women need to incorporate proper diet and nutrition into their daily lifestyle. Diets loaded with fruits, vegetables, whole grains and nuts provide a women's body with the essential nutrients needed to properly supplement the gains achieved during a workout. It is also important the women include ample amount of protein and low-fat dairy products into their diet, as well as foods that contain iron, folic acid and calcium.

Women should avoid or substantially limit the following from their diet:

1. Soft drinks and other beverages that are sugar-sweetened.

2. Alcoholic beverages

3. Foods that are high in saturated fats such as cheese, sausage, baked goods and pizza.

Chapter 5. Bodyweight Training Is Ideal for Women of All Ages

For women who are looking for a workout regimen that is versatile, adaptable and doesn't require equipment or huge time commitments, bodyweight training is an ideal option. Basic bodyweight exercises such as sit-ups, push-ups and crunches are easy to master, and from those basic moves countless variations can be added to spice up workouts. Unlike traditional workout programs, there are countless ways that women can create bodyweight workouts so they never become monotonous or boring. Additionally, bodyweight workouts provide women with a way to improve their fitness without judgment others and these workouts can be done with friends to provide a fun form of motivation.

As with any exercise plan, it is important for women seek expert medical advice from a family doctor or physician. Women should undergo a comprehensive physical to see if there are any physical limitations that need to be kept in mind while engaging in a bodyweight exercise program. With bodyweight training, women can enjoy the benefits of a lean and sculpted body without complicated workout programs, expensive equipment and the use of personal trainers. Ultimately, the sky is the limit with bodyweight training.

Thank You Page

I want to personally thank you for reading my book. I hope you found information in this book useful and I would be very grateful if you could leave your honest review about this book. I certainly want to thank you in advance for doing this.

www.ingramcontent.com/pod-product-compliance
Lightning Source LLC
LaVergne TN
LVHW021746060526
838200LV00052B/3505